KETOGENIC DIET:

The Go-To-Diet for Weight Loss

Disclaimer

The information provided in this book is designed to provide helpful information on the subjects discussed. The author's books are only meant to provide the reader with the basics knowledge of the topic in question, without any warranties regarding whether the reader will, or will not, be able to incorporate and apply all the information provided. Although the writer will make his best effort share her insights, the topic in question is a complex one, and each person needs a different timeframe to fully incorporate new information. Neither this book, nor any of the author's books constitute a promise that the reader will learn anything within a certain timeframe.

Table of Contents

Introduction

If you have been for some time now been thinking of starting your ketogenic diet journey then I urge you to do exactly that. I say this because I believe it is a path that will highly benefit you and that basically includes improving your general health and wellbeing. So many problems that people experience could easily be solved if only we chose ketogenic diet over other types of diets. That could be losing weight, improving mood, headaches etc.

The book will offer the best introduction into the world of low carb revolution, giving you a deeper understanding of what it really is about and also the implementation process. The benefits are diverse and the reason I am so excited to have the opportunity of introducing you to the idea of ketogenic diet. The truth is that our bodies have lost the ability to burn ketones that being fat for energy effectively, because most of our diets are heavy in carbs and sugar. Ketogenic diet is what you need to change all that so you really need to pay close attention to each chapter of the book so that you gain so much.

As an introduction you should know that ketogenic diet is that which allows for the consumption of natural proteins and fats but limits the consumption of carbohydrates. According to research an individual can easily increase their energy and improve health by simply the way they eat or rather what they eat. My emphasis on why a person should try out ketogenic diet is because of its ability to reignite your fat burning engines and impacting profoundly on your longevity and health. The ketogenic diet makes it very effortless for one to lose weight because once the dietary fat is used up a person's system turns to burning the stubborn unhealthy fat for energy.

Am sure you know that the two things that mostly stand out when we talk about maintaining a healthy lifestyle are diet and physical activity. A big part of this book will focus on the idea of diet and you should know everything you eat always has a way of showing on the outside of your body. If you want to feel good and look good then my advice is you need to watch what you eat. Don't be the kind of person who eats to get full but rather to stay healthy.

Chapter One: Understanding The Ketogenic Diet

If you have been looking for a weight loss plan that is effective and safe then ketogenic diet should be your new thing. It is easy to follow and will allow you to lose excess body fat in a short period of time. So what exactly is the ketogenic diet? It is a type of diet that was designed years back and was originally used in treating epilepsy and worked quite well. In defining ketogenic diet you need to know it as a high fat, adequate protein and low carb type of diet. Its effectiveness when it comes to losing weight is seen in the fact that it normally changes the way energy is used in the body and this means the body turns to stored fat for fuel. By following the diet your body reaches a state of ketosis which is what allows for quick weight loss and improved health.

It is what you may have heard people refer to as keto and mainly entails drastically reducing carbohydrate intake and then replacing it with fat. By doing that a person puts their body into a metabolic state called ketosis. This is whereby the body produces ketone bodies when it turns to fat due to lack of carbohydrates and uses them as the main source of energy. Ketosis can only occur when there is limited access to glucose that is always the preferred source of energy for many body cells. With a low carb diet like ketogenic, insulin levels go down and you find that fatty acids are released from fat stores in huge amounts. The fatty acids are then transferred into the liver, oxidized and then transformed into ketone bodies that ultimately provide body energy. Generally, when your body is in ketosis then it means there is higher than normal level of ketone bodies in the blood, lipid energy metabolism is intact and the body begins breaking down body fat for it to fuel all functions. The metabolic change achieved by following a ketogenic diet is very important as it's what improves wellbeing.

The truth is that ketogenic diet is a very simple and also effective way to get lean, strong and healthier. It however requires knowing all of its guidelines, tips and also commonly made mistakes. This will be a way of ensuring that you are always a step ahead and have a deeper understanding of what is required from you. When a person has all that knowledge, they have a chance to lose fat, and at the same time gain muscle. Much of what a person does is limit or restricts the intake of carbohydrate and maximize fat intake. It is always a good idea to know the foods you should or should not eat as a way of maximizing effectiveness. As you start with the ketogenic diet it is essential for you to always plan ahead. One thing you should also note is that what you choose to eat will highly depend on how fast you want to reach ketosis state. The thing is, the more restrictive you are on your carbohydrates then the faster you will enter into ketosis.

Chapter Two: The Main Benefits of Ketogenic Diet

As mention, the ketogenic diet is a very low-carb diet that normally turns a person's body into a fat burning machine. Apart from aiding in weight loss it also comes with potential benefits for health and performance. One of the most admirable and rewarding pursuits in life is that of a healthy lifestyle and ketogenic diet puts you on that track. The popularity of ketogenic diet keeps growing as so many people are now realizing its importance. I want you to learn of its major benefits so that you will have a clearer picture in mind of all that you are in for. Explained below are the benefits:

Fighting Against Cancer

According to research, the ketogenic diet comes in very handy in fighting cancer and this is one of the reasons why it stands out among other forms of diet. One thing about cancer cells is that they normally feed of sugar and this means choosing a diet that eliminates sugar and other carbohydrates puts you on a path to fighting cancer. What you should also note is that our normal body cells can use fat for energy but cancer cells are unable to shift metabolically to using fat. When you introduce the ketogenic diet into your life it will limit the growth and spread of these cancer cells. This happens because with a ketogenic diet, the cancer cells are likely to be starved.

Allows For Quick Weight Loss

There are several reasons why people choose ketogenic diet to help them lose weight and these include the fact that it allows the body to burn excess fat. There is also the fact that it allows the body to get rid of excess water which always adds up to a person's general weight. When you are on a ketogenic diet your energy increases and that means a chance to increase physical activity thus weight loss. You should also know that while on this diet you are likely to feel less hungry and this is because ketone bodies reduce appetite and fat is very satisfying. This means more room for weight loss as you won't struggle with food addiction issues.

Improves Mental Focus

One other thing about the ketogenic diet is that it has the potential of improving your brain function and this allows for improved mental focus. You will also be in a position to avoid big swings in blood sugar and these aspects lead to increased focus and long term concentration. What you may not know is that our brains are over 60% fat by weight and this means the more fat you eat the easier it becomes for it to maintain itself and therefore work to full capacity.

Improves Sleep Apnea

According to studies, sleep apnea is linked to the consumption of grain and ketogenic diet gives you a chance to reduce its intake. Sleep apnea can actually lead to more complications as it interferes with your sleeping habits thus your quality of sleep.

Physical Endurance

Another benefit of ketogenic diet is that it increases a person's physical endurance and this is by giving you a continuous access to energy from stored fats. Normally, the body's supply of stored carbohydrates will last for just some few hours of intense exercise but when depending on fat stores there is a constant access to energy. It therefore means, if one is looking for physical endurance ketogenic diet provides the body with the needed fuel to keep going.

Epilepsy

The ketogenic diet was from the beginning designed as a proven medical therapy for epilepsy. It was mostly used on epileptic children but has recently been tested on adults and gave really good results. The great things about ketogenic diet are that it normally reduces seizures and allows patients to take less anti-epileptic drugs while it still controls the epilepsy.

Stabilizes mood

What ketogenic diet does when it comes to your general mood is that it helps in stabilizing neurotransmitters like serotonin and dopamine and that ultimately results to better mood control.

Chapter Three: Ketogenic Diet Mistakes and Tips

There are a number of mistakes one is likely to make when on their keto program and this may be a real drawback. Knowing these mistakes increases your chances in succeeding especially when trying to lose weight. These mistakes are actually stumbling blocks that may end up compromising your whole diet plan. The truth is that just being able to cut down your carb intake is not enough for you to get into full blown ketosis and also reap all the metabolic benefits of ketogenic diet. You need to be aware of all the commonly made mistakes as this makes it easier for you to avoid them.

1. Obsessing over macros is a mistake because when your full focus is on that you may not be able to fully enhance other aspects of the diet. There is a difference between tracking and obsessing over macros so all you need to do is know the right food and invest in it.

2. Having very high expectations is also another mistake you are likely to make especially for beginners. The ketogenic diet is not magical so exercise patience by doing everything right and you will fully reap the benefits. Having very high expectations may be a reason for you to quit before getting very far. It is more effective and healthy to lose weight long term. The truth is that keto is not a quick fix diet but rather a lifestyle change.

3. It is recommended that you eat proteins but taking too much of it is wrong as it will sabotage your efforts to reach a state of ketosis. It is always said that for every 100g of protein, 56g can be converted to glucose so eating more than needed means the excess will be converted to glucose.

4. There are also those who go for the wrong kinds of fat which is wrong, the idea is not eating much of any kind of fat but the right kind. This therefore calls for you to eat saturated fats, fish oil and monounsaturated fat.

5. You could be tempted to eat processed keto food but that hinders you from achieving the end goal. When following a ketogenic diet then it is all about whole food, actual food and

real food. Preparing and planning for your meals in advance is what allows you to eat the right foods.

6. It is also wrong to not give the diet plan full commitment as ketogenic diet is not for the weak hearted. It requires your dedication, willingness and real determination for you to maximize the benefits.

7. Stop comparing yourself to others when trying to lose weight because someone else's progress is not a determining factor in your success. People gain and lose fat in different areas and at different rates. It is therefore completely wrong to base your success on the progress of another person. As long as you are doing it right just stick to your program and put your focus there.

8. It is clear that it is a low carb diet, so don't make the mistake of eating too many carbs because you won't meet your set goals. This will help you get into a state of ketosis and will have plenty of ketones in your bloodstream thus supplying the brain with enough energy source.

9. Not engaging in physical activity is another major mistake a person is likely to make. It doesn't have to be vigorous because just some few minutes of jogging and walking can have an impact on your general body weight.

10. When on a ketogenic diet there are those who don't take water or enough of it which is a mistake. It is always important for low carb dieters to drink a lot of water for them to stay hydrated. This will help your kidney and liver to process consumed protein and fat.

Chapter Four: Ketogenic Diet Meal Plan

It will take some time for you to get into ketosis and you need to adapt by eating low carb foods for about 7 days. During the 7 days there will be short periods of fatigue, sluggishness, headaches and sometime might experience gastrointestinal problems or 'keto flu' as you get used to it. Most of these issues can be corrected by taking the right electrolyte and you shouldn't be much worried about the caloric restriction. As your body begins to regulate your appetite it is when you will lose weight because your addiction to processed foods and sugar will reduce; that's why it isn't recommended that you restrict your caloric intake during this meal plan.

The ketogenic meal plan is designed to help you get a balanced diet that ensures you eat healthy meals that address satiation and provides fiber and plenty protein intake. With ketogenic diet you won't need to sacrifice muscle for your body to burn fat and after weight loss you will have a body shape that you desire. This diet will also help you lose significant amount of water as your body will convert the carbs to glycogen, which will be stored in water within the liver and muscles. When your body uses up the stored glycogen, your body will automatically remove this water; this will help you lose extra weight and it will also reduce bloating. Take into account that every person has different needs and you are also required to adjust your meal plan as you start losing weight because your needs will change. Keep your recipes to be simple because this will help you to enjoy and stick to the meal plan. Some of the things you should also remember include:

1. Breakfast should contain non-starchy vegetables, which should be around 16g of carbs, some fat and a protein.
2. When it comes to lunch; avoid sugar, milk, starchy vegetables, yogurt and fruits and make sure the carbohydrates you take from non-starchy vegetables are less than16g. One of the most convenient meals to take for lunch is salad.
3. For dinner, choose foods rich in proteins such as fish, chicken, pork, turkey, beef or seafood. You should also include non-starchy vegetables like green beans, broccoli, red bell pepper

or Brussels sprouts; make sure carbohydrates content is less than 16g.
4. Choose snacks that contain less than 7g of carbohydrates but should have enough of protein and fat.

When you are looking for ingredients, make sure you get them in their most organic or natural form and without unnecessary additives.

DAY ONE: MONDAY

Keto Scrambled Eggs

Time: 20 minutes

Serving(s): 1

Ingredients:

- 3 large eggs
- 1 tablespoon unsalted butter
- A pinch freshly ground pepper
- A pinch coarse salt

Directions:

1. Start by beating the eggs with a fork.
2. In a medium non-stick skillet, melt the butter over low heat and then add the egg mixture.
3. Use a heatproof flexible spatula to lightly pull the eggs to the center of the skillet and heat until the liquid parts run out.
4. Now, cook while repeatedly using the spatula to move the eggs for approximately 3 minutes or until they are set.
5. Season with salt and pepper, serve while still hot.

Nutritional Facts per Serving: Calories 318, Fat 26.3g, Carbohydrates 1.8g and Protein 17.4g.

Tasty Ginger Beef

Time: 30 minutes

Serving(s): 1

Ingredients:

- 2 cut in strips of sirloin steaks
- 1 clove of crushed garlic
- 2 small diced tomatoes
- 1 small diced onion
- 4 tablespoons apple cider vinegar
- 1 teaspoon ground ginger
- 1 tablespoon Olive oil
- Salt and pepper

Directions:

1. In a large skillet, heat the olive oil and place the steak over medium-heat until brown and make sure that both sides are well-seared. Add the garlic, onion, and tomatoes and continue cooking.
2. Stir the salt, pepper and ginger into the vinegar in a bowl and then add the mixture to the pan, stirring frequently to combine.
3. Cover the pan, turn heat to low and allow the mixture to simmer; make sure that the liquids have evaporated completely.
4. Serve and enjoy!

Nutritional Facts per Serving: Calories 208, Fat 8g, Carbohydrates 3g and Protein 31g.

Creamy Spinach with Salmon

Time: 30 minutes

Serving(s): 1

Ingredients:

- 1 small salmon or trout fillet
- 1-2 tablespoon coconut oil, extra virgin olive oil or ghee
- 1 tablespoon heavy whipping cream or coconut milk
- 1 serving Hollandaise sauce
- ½ large packet fresh or frozen spinach
- Freshly ground black pepper
- A pinch of salt to taste

Directions:

1. Preheat the oven to 400 degrees F.
2. In a baking tray, place the salmon and sprinkle with half of the coconut oil, olive oil or ghee; season with salt and pepper to taste, place in the oven and cook for about 30 minutes.
3. In the meantime, set up the creamy spinach. Wash the spinach and pat dry with a paper towel or place in a salad spinner to get rid of any excess water.
4. Use half of the coconut oil, olive oil or ghee to grease a skillet and heat over medium-high heat. Put in the spinach and continue cooking for 3-6 minutes while mixing and then season with salt to taste.
5. Add the coconut milk or heavy whipping cream. Remove from heat and set aside. In the meantime, prepare the Hollandaise sauce.
6. Now, remove salmon from the oven and reserve for 5 minutes
7. On a serving plate, place the creamed spinach and top with the baked salmon.

8. Pour the mixture over the Hollandaise sauce. Serve and enjoy!

Nutritional Facts per Serving: Calories 290, Carbohydrates3.7g, Fat 72.6g, Fiber 2.8g and Protein 34g.

DAY TWO: TUESDAY

Chocolate with Chia Pudding

Time: 15 minutes

Serving(s): 1

Ingredients:

- ¼ cup, whole or ground Chia seeds
- ½ cup of water or almond milk
- 1 tablespoon Erythritol or other healthy low-carb sweetener, powdered
- ¼ cup heavy whipping cream or coconut milk
- 1 tablespoon raw cacao powder, unsweetened
- 5-10 drops Stevia extract
- Top with: Extra dark chocolate (no less than 85% cocoa solids) or ½ tablespoon raw cocoa nibs
- *Optional*: ¼ teaspoon add cinnamon or cayenne pepper

Directions:

1. Combine the coconut milk, chia seeds, cacao powder, water, stevia and Erythritol. If you want a smoother texture, you can place the ingredients in a blender and process until smooth.
2. Leave it for about 12-15 minutes or if possible place it in the fridge overnight. Once it's ready, top with the cocoa ribs just before you serve.

Nutritional Facts per Serving: Calories 329, Carbs: 6.3g, Fiber 14.9g, Fat 26.6g, Protein 9.5g, Magnesium 63mg and Potassium 364mg.

Lunch

Peri Peri Chicken, Spinach with Bacon Salad

Time: 30 minutes

Serving(s): 1

Ingredients:

- 2 cups baby spinach
- 1/3 if large and ½ if small avocado
- ½ chicken breast
- 1 tablespoon Peri Peri Sauce
- 1-piece low sodium bacon

Directions:

1. In a pan, place the bacon and cook until it becomes crispy and brown; set aside the bacon fat.
2. Meanwhile, chop the chicken breast into even pieces. Add the slices of chicken into the bacon fat and cook one side for 1 minute. Toss it and then fry for 5-7 minutes.
3. Meanwhile, cut the avocado and bacon into small pieces. Place avocado and spinach into a large bowl and then add the sliced bacon and Peri Peri sauce.

Nutritional Facts per Serving: Calories 330, Carbs 10g, Fat 16g, Protein 36g and Fiber 6g.

Coconut Shrimps with Avocados

Time: 25 minutes

Serving(s): 1

Ingredients:

- 1 cup of shrimps
- ½ tablespoon of organic peanut butter
- ½ avocados
- 1 teaspoon of coconut Shredded
- 1 tablespoon of lite coconut milk
- Sriracha hot sauce

Directions:

1. Using olive oil sprayer, spray a nonstick pan on medium temperature and then pour the peanut butter, coconut milk and Sriracha hot sauce.
2. Place the shrimps and cook until shrimps are pink or for 3-5 minutes.
3. Cut the avocado in cubes and place it on a plate and then top with shrimps and drizzle with shredded coconut.

Nutritional Facts per Serving: Calories 250, Fat 12g, Carbs 7g, Protein 24g and Fibers 4g.

DAY THREE: WEDNESDAY

Keto Breakfast

Time: 25 minutes

Serving(s): 2

Ingredients:

- 5 thin slices or 3 regular bacon
- 1 large egg, free-range or organic
- ½ average avocado
- a pinch freshly ground black pepper
- 2 large Portobello mushrooms
- 1 tablespoon butter or ghee
- Salt to taste
- Fresh herbs for garnish
- Recommended replacements that have the same net carb effect:
  - Instead of mushroom you can use 2 cups of cooked spinach
  - Instead of bacon you can use 1 grain-free sausage
  - Instead of avocado you can use 2 oz. cheese like cheddar

Directions:

1. Start by pan-roasting the mushrooms. Heat half of the ghee or butter on a non-stick skillet over medium-low heat and then place the mushrooms, drizzle them with pepper and sea salt.
2. Cook until tender or for about 10 minutes. Some water will be released by the mushrooms, try frying the egg on a different butter-greased skillet together with the bacon.

Nutritional Facts per Serving: Calories 489, Carbs 6.6g, Protein 19.5g, Fat 41.3g, Fiber 8.9g, Potassium 1307mg and Magnesium 43mg

Lunch

Salmon and Avocado

Time: 30 minutes

Serving(s): 2

Ingredients:

- 1 large or 2 small-medium avocado seed removed
- 2 small Salmon fillets
- ¼ cup Crème fraîche, soured cream or mayonnaise
- 1 small, finely chopped white onion
- 1-2 tablespoons freshly chopped dill
- 2 tablespoons fresh lemon juice
- 1 tablespoon coconut oil or ghee
- ¼ teaspoon or more salt; to taste
- Freshly ground black pepper; to taste
- Lemon wedges for garnish
- *Note:* Always try to get ingredients in their most organic and natural form and without any additives.

Directions:

1. Preheat the oven to about 400 degrees.
2. Line a parchment paper on a baking tray and then add the salmon filets. Sprinkle with olive oil or melted ghee, add salt

and pepper to taste and fresh lemon juice (1 tablespoon). Cook in the oven for about 25 minutes.

3. Once done, transfer from oven and set aside for about 10 minutes so that it can cool.
4. Chop the salmon fillets with a folk and throw away the skin. Combine with finely sliced onions, finely sliced dill and crème fraîche, soured cream or mayonnaise.
5. Drizzle more lemon juice and season with salt and pepper. Scoop the flesh part of the avocado but make sure you leave about an inch of the avocado flesh. Slice and place in a bowl with salmon and then mix well to combine.
6. Take the avocado with salmon mixture and fill each avocado halve; add more lemon.
7. Serve and enjoy!

Nutritional Facts per Serving: Calories 463, Carbohydrates6.4g, Fiber 7.5g, Protein27g, Fat34.6g, Potassium 1122mg and magnesium 75mg

Dinner

Keto Stir Fry

Time: 20 minutes

Serving(s): 3

Ingredients:

- 1 tablespoon of coconut oil
- 1/2 medium Spanish onion
- 5 medium brown mushrooms
- 2 kale leaves
- 1/2 cup broccoli
- 1/2 medium red pepper

- 300gof ground beef
- 1 tablespoon of Chinese five Spices
- 1 tablespoon of cayenne pepper

Directions:

1. Start by chopping the broccoli, onion, kale and red pepper and then chop the mushrooms. Heat the coconut oil in a large skillet on medium-high heat, add onions and cook for approximately 1 minute.
2. Add other vegetables and cook for another 2 minutes stirring often.
3. Reduce the heat to medium, add the beef and spices then cook for about 2 minutes.
4. Cover the pan and let it cook for about 10 minutes or until the beef is browned.

Nutritional Facts per Serving: Calories 307, Carbohydrates 7g, Fat 18g and Protein 29g

DAY FOUR: THURSDAY

Raspberry Protein Shake

Time: 5 minutes

Serving(s): 1

Ingredients:

- 77g of raspberries
- 24g of natural peanut butter
- 1 cup of almond milk
- 1 scoop of strawberry protein powder
- ¼teaspoon of ginger
- ¼teaspoon of cinnamon
- 1 tablespoon of ground coffee; optional

Directions:

- Place the all the ingredients in your blender and puree until smooth.
- Serve and enjoy!

Nutritional Facts per Serving: Calories 319, Fat 15g, Carbs 10g, Protein 28g, Fiber 7g and Sodium 264mg.

Cobb Salad

Time: 25 minutes

Serving(s): 1

Ingredients:

For the dressing:

- 1 tablespoon Olive oil
- 1 tablespoon Organic apple cider vinegar
- 1 teaspoon lemon juice
- 1 teaspoon Dijon Mustard
- Salt and pepper to taste
- Garlic (a little bit); optional

For the Cobb Salad:

- Extra virgin olive oil cooking spray
- 2 hard-boiled eggs
- 100g ham
- 30g Blue cheese
- 4 Cherry tomatoes
- 2 cups, coarsely chopped Romaine lettuce
- ½ diced avocado
- 2 slices Turkey bacon

Directions:

1. Start by hard boiling the eggs either with a regular method or with a pre-programmed steamer. Place the olive oil in a non-stick pan and then add diced ham and heat for about 5 minutes.

2. In the bottom of a bowl, place the lettuce and then slice the hard boiled eggs
3. Arrange halved blue cheese, cherry tomatoes, ham, avocadoes, turkey bacon and eggs in rows and then spread the dressing evenly.

Nutritional Facts per Serving: Calories 370, Carbohydrates 7g, Fat 27g and Proteins 46g

Dinner

Paprika Chicken

Time: 1 hour

Serving(s): 4

Ingredients:

- 8-12 chicken drumsticks; with bone and skin
- 1 medium white onion
- 1 cup chicken stock or water
- 1 tablespoon Paprika
- 2 tablespoons Ghee
- ¼ cup soured cream or more coconut milk
- ¼ cup coconut milk or heavy whipping cream
- 1 medium red pepper
- Freshly ground black pepper
- ½ teaspoon salt; to taste
- *Optional*: You can serve with about 5 cups cauli-rice

Directions:

1. Use a paper towel to pat dry the chicken and season with salt and pepper.
2. Using a small amount of ghee, grease a Dutch oven or a large soup pot. When it is hot, put the chicken and heat over a medium-high heat until all sides are browned.
3. Add the water or chicken stock and bring to a simmer. Cover it and then lower heat and begin cooking for about 30 minutes.
4. When done, remove the chicken using tongs and set aside in a bowl. If you like you can slice the meat off the bone
5. In the meantime, finely chop the onion and then halve, remove seed and cut the red pepper. Grease another skillet with the remaining ghee, add onions and heat until fragrant and browned. Place the red pepper lice and continue cooking for an additional 5 minutes.
6. Into the pot with chicken stock, add the pepper and onion and then followed by the paprika. Remove from heat and place in a blender, pulse until smooth.
7. Put back on the oven; add the sour cream and heavy whipping cream. Add chicken in the pot with sauce and continue cooking for approximately 5 minutes.

Nutritional Facts per Serving: Calories 714, Carbohydrates 9.8g, Protein 27.2g, Fiber 5.3g, Fat 61.2g, Magnesium 65mg and Potassium 1018mg

DAY FIVE: FRIDAY

Coffee Protein Shake

Time: 10 minutes

Serving(s): 1

Ingredients:

- 1 scoop Vanilla Iso-Flex Isolate Protein Powder
- ¼ cup Greek yogurt
- 1 shot Espresso
- 1 pinch Cinnamon
- 1 pinch Stevia
- Ice cubes (5)

Directions:

1. Prepare your coffee.
2. Place all the ingredients, making sure that the protein powder comes last and process until smooth.

Nutritional Facts per Serving: Calories 169, Fat 1g, Carbohydrates 3g and Protein 35g

Egg Muffin Cup

Time: 35 minutes

Serving(s): 6

Ingredients:

- 6 slices of nitrate free shaved turkey
- 6 eggs
- ½ cup of sliced spinach
- Mozzarella cheese light
- 3 tablespoons of red pepper
- 2 tablespoons of red Onion, finely chopped
- Salt and pepper; to taste
- Fresh Basil; optional

Directions:

1. Preheat the oven to 350 degrees
2. Chop the red onion, spinach, basil and red pepper and grate the mozzarella cheese.
3. Use an olive oil spray to spray a nonstick muffin tin.
4. Cover the piece of turkey gently in one muffin cup and let it rest on the sides and the bottom of the tin so that it can make a larger cup.
5. Whisk the eggs in a small bowl and add it into the turkey cups followed by a little bit of chopped red pepper, red onion, cheese and spinach.
6. Add a little bit of fresh basil and some salt and fresh grinded pepper onto the eggs.
7. Place the muffin tins in the oven and then bake for about 15 minutes if you want a harder yolk or 10 if you prefer a runny

one. Remember that egg muffins will take a bit longer to cook if you take it out of the oven.

Nutritional Facts per Serving: Calories95, Fat6g, Carbohydrates2g, Protein9g and Sodium 200mg

Dinner

Low-Carb Frittata

Time: 20 minutes

Serving(s): 4

Ingredients:

- 1 tablespoon coconut oil
- 4 eggs
- 3 leaves Kale
- 300g fatty ground beef or any meat you prefer and add bacon
- 4 mushrooms
- 1 teaspoon Paprika
- ½ green pepper
- ½ red pepper
- 200g goat cheese; choose one that is low in carb, low in protein and high in fat
- 1 teaspoon garlic powder
- 1 teaspoon curry powder

Directions:

1. Chop the mushrooms, kale, red pepper and green pepper into small cubes.

2. Place the coconut oil in a skillet and heat it; cook the vegetables. Once done, add grounded beef and mix well until browned. Evenly spread the ingredients in the pan.
3. Whisk the eggs with spices and then gently pour it onto the vegetables mixture.
4. Drizzle the goat cheese at the top of the pan and cover the pan until cheese is bubbling and eggs are cooked; this will take about 5 minutes.

Nutritional Facts per Serving: Calories 490, Fat 40g, Carbohydrates 5g, Fibers 1.5g and Protein 25g

DAY SIX: SATURDAY

Chorizo Breakfast Casserole

Time: 1 hour

Serving(s): 10

Ingredients:

- 16 Oz ground chorizo
- 1 small onion
- 1 bunch spinach
- 12 eggs
- 12 tablespoons of heavy cream
- 1 teaspoon of onion powder, garlic powder, pepper and salt
- 1 small green pepper
- Cheddar (8 Oz)
- Cherry tomatoes (9 Oz)

Directions:

1. Place the spinach in the microwave and cook. Chop or crush the chorizo and then cook in a pan until browned. When done place in a large bowl.
2. Cut the green pepper and onion; cook in the same pan and place in a large bowl. Add the spinach to the same bowl.
3. Combine together the heavy cream, eggs and spices.
4. Place the cheese to the bowl and mix well and then add the egg mixture and stir well before transferring it to a greased casserole bowl. If you prefer you can add the cherry tomatoes.
5. Preheat the oven at 350 F and cook for 50 minutes.

Nutritional Facts per Serving: Calories 362, Fat 28, Carbohydrates 7, Fiber 2 and Protein 24

Lunch

Avocado with Egg Salad

Time: 40 minutes

Serving(s): 2

Ingredients:

- 4 large, free-range or organic eggs
- 1 large avocado
- 2 cloves, crushed garlic
- ½ cup full-fat yogurt or soured cream or ¼ cup mayonnaise
- 4 cups mixed lettuce such as arugula, lamb lettuce, etc.
- 2 teaspoons Dijon mustard
- Salt and pepper to taste
- Optional: fresh herbs, extra virgin olive oil and chives for garnish

Directions:

1. Start by filling a small saucepan with water, making sure it reaches ¾ full and add 1-2 pinches of salt and bring to a boil.
2. Use your hand or even a spoon to dip each egg carefully in and out of the boiling water. The salt and dipping of eggs in and out will help prevent the eggs from cracking. Dip for approximately 10 minutes.
3. When done, transfer the eggs to a bowl filled with cold water and when they are chilled, peel off the shells.
4. Mix the Dijon mustard, soured cream and crushed garlic then season with salt and pepper.

5. Pat dry with a paper towel or use a salad spinner to clean and drain the greens and place them in a serving bowl. Deseed peel and cut the avocado and then add on top of the greens.
6. Put in the quartered eggs and season with salt and pepper.

Nutritional Facts per Serving: Calories 436, Carbohydrates 6.1g, Protein 17g, Fat 36.3g, Fiber 7.6g, Magnesium 60mg, Potassium 875mg

Dinner

Meatza

Time: 30 minutes

Serving(s): 4

Ingredients:

- 20 Oz ground beef
- 2 large eggs
- 4 Oz Mozzarella cheese
- ½ cup Cheddar cheese, shredded
- ½ cup Pizza sauce
- 28 slices Pepperoni
- Salt, pepper and garlic powder; to taste

Directions:

1. Combine together the ground beef, eggs and seasoning.
2. Place the mixture into a cast iron skillet so that it can form a pizza crust then cook until meat is ready at 400 degrees; this will take about 15 minutes.

3. When done remove the crust and then add cheese, sauce and toppings and cook again until cheese is fully melted.

Nutritional Facts per Serving: Calories 610, Fat 45, Carbohydrates 3, Fiber 1, Protein 44

DAY SEVEN: SUNDAY

Pesto Scrambled Eggs

Time: 30 minutes

Serving(s): 2

Ingredients:

- 3 large, free-range or organic eggs
- 1 tablespoon, grass-fed butter or ghee
- 1 tablespoon Pesto
- 2 tablespoon Crème fraîche, creamed coconut milk or soured cream
- Salt and freshly ground black pepper; to taste

Directions:

1. In a mixing bowl, whisk the eggs with a pinch of pepper and salt, use a folk or a whisk to stir well.
2. Put the egg mixture in the skillet and then add ghee or butter; cook on low heat while stirring continuously. Add the pesto and stir well to combine.
3. Transfer from heat, add crème fraîche and mix well with the eggs mixture. This will help the eggs to retain a creamy texture and stay cool.
4. Transfer to a serving plate and top with sliced avocado.

Nutritional Facts per Serving: Calories 467, Fiber 0.7g, carbohydrates 2.6g, Protein 20.4g, Fat 41.5g, Magnesium 26mg and Potassium 327mg.

Taco Salad

Time: 25 minutes

Serving(s): 4

Ingredients:

- 32 Oz ground pork
- 9 Oz Cheddar cheese, shredded
- 12 tablespoons sour cream
- 12 tablespoons Salsa
- 6 Romaine leaves
- 6 teaspoons McCormick taco seasoning
- Cayenne pepper; to taste

Directions:

1. Place the pork in a skillet and cook until it is browned.
2. When done, add the taco seasoning and other extra spices and then cook until it is incorporated.
3. Once ready, let it cool then distribute it into 6 containers.
4. Top each container with cheese. Put salsa and sour cream in a prep bowl and then saran wrap it.
5. Put into the container the Romaine Lettuce.

Nutritional Facts per Serving: Calories 647, Fat 51, Carbohydrates 5, Fiber 1, Protein 38

Keto Chili

Time: 6 hours 30 minutes

Serving(s): 8

Ingredients:

- 8 thick cut bacon
- 2 lbs. or 32 oz. ground pork
- 1 medium onion yellow onion
- 6 oz. tomato paste
- 1 can tomatoes, diced and drained
- 3 small peppers green pepper
- 1 pack McCormick original chili seasoning
- Salt, pepper and onion powder, garlic powder, cayenne pepper; to taste

Directions:

1. Cut peppers and onions and put them in Crockpot.
2. Meanwhile, place pork, salt and pepper in a pan and then cook until the pork is browned. Let it cool and add in the Crockpot followed by drained tomatoes.
3. Put in the tomato paste and then followed by the seasoning packet.
4. Cook on low heat for 6 hours.

Nutritional Facts per Serving: Calories 492, Fat 35, Carbohydrates 13, Fiber 4 and Protein 31

LOW-CARB SNACKS AND ADDITIONS

Keto Scrambled Eggs. As from the previous recipe, Keto Scrambled Eggs can be served with bacon and coffee (with adding almond milk to the coffee).

Spinach Salad. Place 2 slices of chicken breast or any other cold meat and a handful of spinach and then spray with olive oil. Put in one teaspoon of apple cider vinegar, one teaspoon of parmesan cheese and then drizzle with almonds. Serve and enjoy!

Apple with warm almond butter. This snack should be taken as a mini treat and all you are required to do is to dip apple in warm almond butter.

Cheese, Broccoli with Stuffed Chicken Breast. This is a pretty useful snack if you don't have time to cook. In this recipe you are supposed to include cheese and broccoli because they contain fewer carbohydrates, you can also include spinach or feta.

Egg Muffins. It is a remarkable snack because you can carry it wherever you go. They also contain fewer carbohydrates and are lean.

Mixed nuts. Take a handful of nuts and seeds and it can either be raw or cooked with sea salt. Some of them with their net carb per serving include sunflower seeds - 3.2 g, pecans - 1.2 g, walnuts - 2 g, pumpkin seeds - 1.3 g, almonds - 2.7 g, macadamias - 1.5 g, brazil nuts - 1.4 g, hazelnuts - 2 g and pine nuts - 2.7 g. it is also recommended that you soak the nuts.

Half avocado and pink Himalayan salt.

Crispy bacon slices. You should make this in advance and store in the fridge.

Coffee with coconut milk, almond milk or cream or you can even take low carb cappuccino.

Salted hardboiled egg. One hardboiled egg; add Himalayan salt to taste.

Chicken cracklings or pork cracklings/rinds instead of chips. You should also avoid products with additives.

Avoid taking peanut butter and instead take other nuts like Pecan butter with two tablespoons of homemade coconut and two to three celery sticks.

Coconut oil can also be taken as a quick fat burning snack and all you are required to do is store one tablespoon in the fridge.

Take fresh or frozen berries and some of them with their net carb include ½ cup blackberries - 3.1 g, ½ cup raspberries - 3.3 g, ½ cup strawberries - 4.1 g or ¼ cup blueberries - 4.5 g).

Chapter Five: Other Factors to Consider in Weight Loss

Apart from ketogenic diet there are also some aspects to consider that will help in accelerating your weight loss. These are just basic things that you should always have in mind and I believe will be highly effective. They are as highlighted below:

Stress Reduction

It is known that stress levels and weight gain are closely related because with increased stress your level of physical activity reduces and appetite pattern changes. To allow yourself to lose weight easily then work on your stress to avoid emotional eating and create room for weight loss.

Eating All Meals

Skipping meals especially breakfast is never a weight loss solution as all one needs to focus on is eating the right food at the right time. When you skip meals it means you will eat more than enough on your next meal because of excess hunger. This is much about eating more calories than you actually would have. Another thing to note is that by skipping meals, your body holds on to fat, metabolism is depressed and you can lose muscles.

Getting Quality Sleep

To complement your ketogenic diet, I advise you to make an effort of maintaining healthy sleeping habits. There are situations when a person could be physically active and follows a healthy diet plan but is still not losing weight. Chances are that you are not getting enough sleep or quality sleep which normally affects the leptin and ghrelin levels known to be the body's checks and balances and responsible for stimulating and suppressing appetite. Leptin suppresses appetite while ghrelin stimulates appetite. Lack of enough sleep leads to a drop in your leptin levels while it increases your ghrelin levels which means you are likely to crave for sugary and high carb foods.

Drinking Water

 A person should also be in the habit of drinking enough water as it plays a huge role during weight loss. What it does is that it boosts metabolism, cleanses the body and suppresses appetite. With enough water the body won't need to retain excess water which is what contributes to increased weight. Another good thing about drinking water is that it has the potential of boosting metabolism.

Exercising

The best lifestyle change to make when you want to lose weight is adapting to a healthy eating habit and being physically active. A person should therefore make exercising a regular routine for them to easily burn calories and also build muscles. You don't have to start out big because even just some few minutes of moderate exercises allows for weight loss.

Conclusion

It is my hope that this book was able to help you understand what Ketogenic diet is and most importantly enlightened you on how it can be applied to achieve quick weight loss. It is always a struggle for many people who are overweight but I assure you with willingness and commitment you can easily achieve the body shape and size you desire. Each chapter of the book gave you specific information that I believe will be of great help and puts you on a path to living a healthy and happy lifestyle. It is therefore your responsibility to put into practice all that you have learnt for you to realize that all efforts put into having this book was all worth it.

Additional Bonus

1-page 7-Day Meal Plan

Day	Meals	Notes
Day 1	**Breakfast** > Keto Scrambled Eggs **Lunch** > Tasty Ginger Beef **Dinner** > Creamy Spinach with Salmon	
Day 2	**Breakfast** > Chocolate with Chia Pudding **Lunch** > Peri Peri Chicken, Spinach with Bacon Salad **Dinner** > Coconut Shrimps with Avocados	
Day 3	**Breakfast** > Keto Breakfast **Lunch** > Salmon and Avocado **Dinner** > Keto Stir Fry	
Day 4	**Breakfast** > Raspberry Protein Shake **Lunch** > Cobb Salad **Dinner** > Paprika Chicken	
Day 5	**Breakfast** > Coffee Protein Shake **Lunch** > Egg Muffin Cup **Dinner** > Low-Carb Frittata	
Day 6	**Breakfast** > Chorizo Breakfast Casserole **Lunch** > Avocado with Egg Salad **Dinner** > Meatza	
Day 7	**Breakfast** > Pesto Scrambled Eggs **Lunch** > Taco Salad **Dinner** > Keto Chili	
Additional meals / notes: